WHY GLASSES?

Why Glasses?

The Story of Vision

By George John Sands, M. D.

Illustrated by Rov André

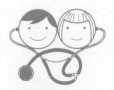

Published by

MEDICAL BOOKS FOR CHILDREN

LERNER PUBLICATIONS COMPANY

MINNEAPOLIS, MINNESOTA

© 1960 by Lerner Publications Company

All rights reserved—no part of this book
may be reproduced in any form without
permission in writing from the publisher,
except by a reviewer who wishes to quote
brief passages in connection with a review
written for inclusion in magazine or news-
paper.

International Copyright Secured. Printed in U.S.A.

Library of Congress Catalog Card Number: 60-16744

Third Printing 1962
Fourth Printing 1964
Fifth Printing 1966
Sixth Printing 1967
Seventh Printing 1968

TABLE OF CONTENTS

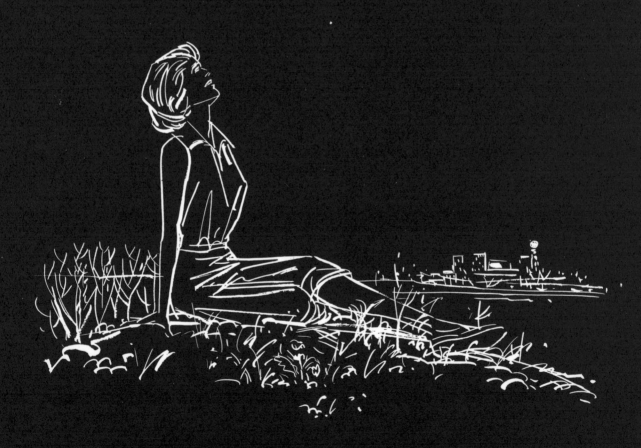

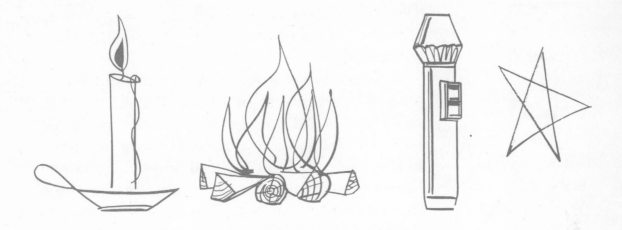

1 OUR EYES SEE LIGHT

If you were outside on a very dark night, when the moon and the stars were hiding behind clouds, you would not be able to see.

If you were inside on a sunny day, but your house had no lights or windows or doors to let the sun in, you would not be able to see.

You would need a candle or a flashlight or a fire burning or light from a star in order to see.

Without light, everything would be invisible.

It doesn't matter where the light comes from. As long as there *is* light, that light can be reflected or bounced off people and things so that our eyes can see them.

Our eyes see light. Light travels in waves that move faster than automobiles, trains, jets or rockets. Light speeds along at

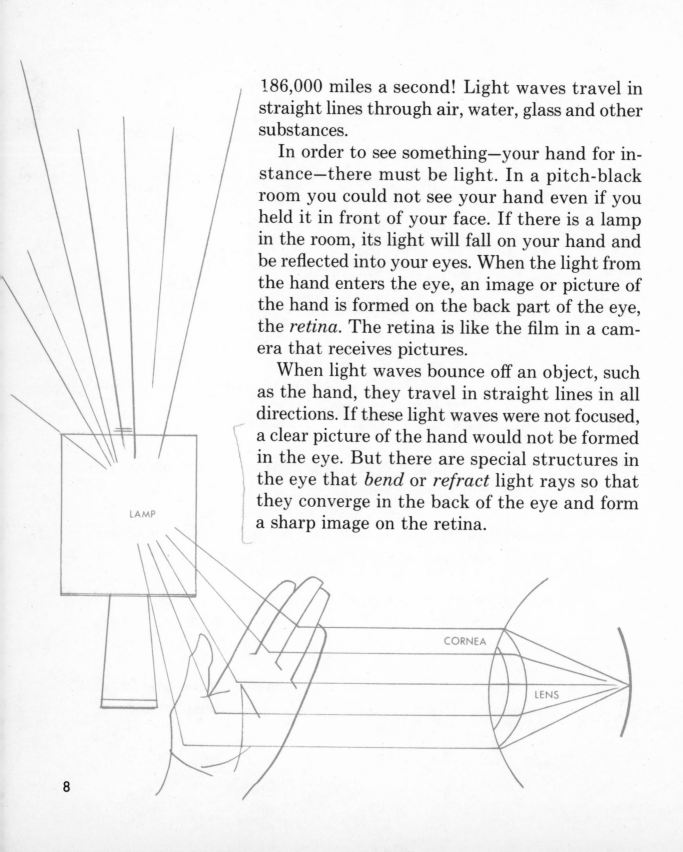

186,000 miles a second! Light waves travel in straight lines through air, water, glass and other substances.

In order to see something—your hand for instance—there must be light. In a pitch-black room you could not see your hand even if you held it in front of your face. If there is a lamp in the room, its light will fall on your hand and be reflected into your eyes. When the light from the hand enters the eye, an image or picture of the hand is formed on the back part of the eye, the *retina*. The retina is like the film in a camera that receives pictures.

When light waves bounce off an object, such as the hand, they travel in straight lines in all directions. If these light waves were not focused, a clear picture of the hand would not be formed in the eye. But there are special structures in the eye that *bend* or *refract* light rays so that they converge in the back of the eye and form a sharp image on the retina.

LAMP

CORNEA

LENS

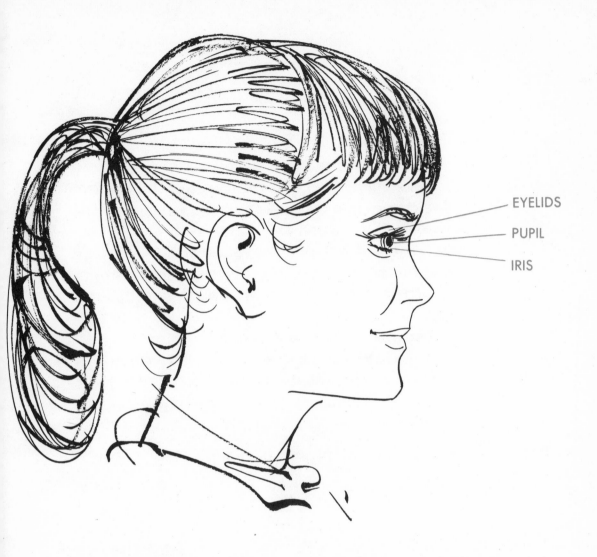

EYELIDS

PUPIL

IRIS

II HOW THE EYES WORK

Structures that Assist the Eye

The eye is round like a ball. At its top and bottom are eyelids which can be shut tight to keep out dirt. The eyelids are more than protective covers. They help mop up the surface of the eyeball with tears secreted by the tear or *lacrimal glands*. The eyelashes help brush harmful objects away from the eye. The eye can be moved up, down and sideways by muscles.

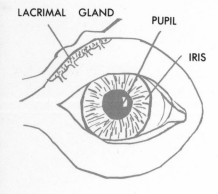

LACRIMAL GLAND

PUPIL

IRIS

The Coats of the Eye

The eyeball is not a perfect sphere because it has a slight bulge in front called the *cornea*. The cornea makes up 1/6 of the surface of the eyeball. The other 5/6 of the wall of the eyeball, the "white" of the eye, consists of a tough coat or membrane, the *sclera*. Light cannot enter the sclera because it is thick and opaque. Light can enter the cornea because it is thin and transparent like a bubble.

The cornea is very sensitive, and when dirt and eyelashes get in the eye they cause pain. The eyelids blink automatically to protect this delicate window from injury.

The Focusing Parts of the Eye

Beneath the cornea is a space filled with fluid or *aqueous*. This space is divided into front and back rooms—the *anterior* and *posterior chambers*—by a colored curtain called the *iris*. The iris appears blue or brown depending upon the amount of pigment or color it contains. The iris is shaped like a ring. The hole in the ring is the *pupil*. The iris controls the size of the pupil to let in light.

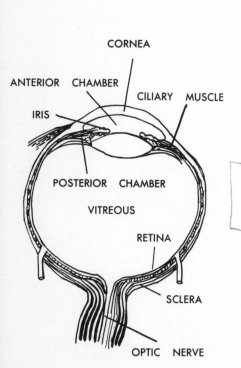

CORNEA

ANTERIOR CHAMBER

CILIARY MUSCLE

IRIS

POSTERIOR CHAMBER

VITREOUS

RETINA

SCLERA

OPTIC NERVE

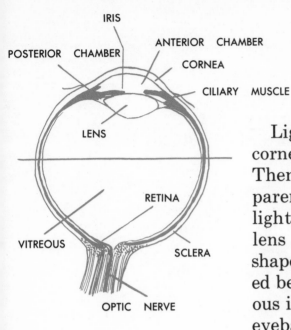

IRIS

ANTERIOR CHAMBER

POSTERIOR CHAMBER

CORNEA

CILIARY MUSCLE

LENS

RETINA

VITREOUS

SCLERA

OPTIC NERVE

Light entering the eye passes through the cornea, the anterior chamber and the pupil. Then it reaches the *lens*. The lens is transparent and elastic. It is important in bringing light rays to a sharp focus on the retina. The lens gets its name from lentil because it is shaped like a lentil seed or a pea. It is suspended between the iris and the *vitreous*. The vitreous is a jelly-like material that helps keep the eyeball round. A band of fibers connects the lens to the *ciliary muscles* which are anchored to the wall of the eyeball.

Because the lens is elastic, it can become round or flat depending upon how much it is pulled by the ciliary muscles. They help the lens change its shape by *contracting* and *relaxing*. Try looking at your finger when you hold it up in front of your nose. Do you feel the ciliary muscles contract? Now look at your finger when you hold your arm out in front of you as far as you can. Do you feel the ciliary muscles relax?

When the eyes look at an object that is near by, the ciliary muscles contract. And the lens springs into a thicker shape. When the eyes look at a distant object, the ciliary muscles re-

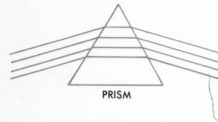

PRISM

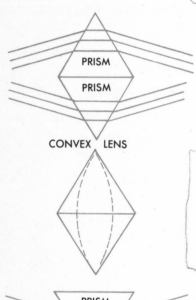

PRISM
PRISM

CONVEX LENS

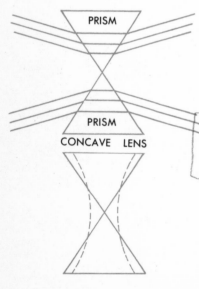

PRISM

PRISM
CONCAVE LENS

lax. And the lens flattens out. The change in shape of the lens in order to focus is called *accommodation.*

The lens bends light just the way a *prism* does. A prism is a solid piece of glass that looks like a triangle from the end. Light rays are bent when they go into the prism and again when they come out. All rays are bent toward the bottom of the prism.

If two prisms are put together with the bases of the triangles touching each other, the light rays are converged to one spot or focus. If the edges of the prisms are rounded off, a *convex lens* is formed. The lens of the eye is convex. Burning glass is a convex lens that converges the sun's rays. The heat produced is so intense that fire can result.

If two prisms are put together with the tops of the triangles touching each other, the light rays are divergent or bent away from one another. This is how a *concave lens* is formed.

The cornea, lens and vitreous all bend light so that the image of an object can be focused on the retina.

The retina is the innermost lining of the eyeball. It is more than just a film to catch pictures. In the retina are over 100 million tiny

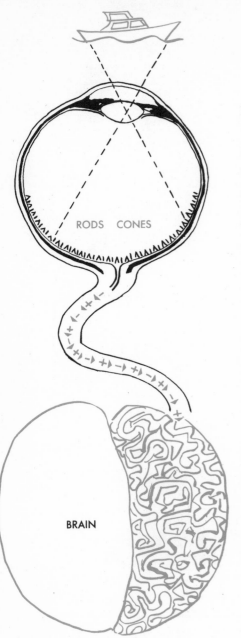

nerve cells, called rods and cones, that contain chemicals which react to light. Each rod and cone is connected to a nerve fiber thinner than thread. The nerve fibers join together into a large nerve, called the *optic nerve,* which leads right to the brain. The image of an object that falls on the retina is upside down just the way an object appears upside down when seen through a camera. The brain turns the image right-side up.

When light falls on the sensitive rods and cones of the retina, a chemical change occurs in these cells. This chemical change starts "impulses" moving along the nerve pathways to the brain.

The nerve impulses are like electric signals that send messages. The brain receives the impulses and is able to translate them into a picture that we can see and understand. We do not know the exact way that the brain does this. We do know that the result is what we call vision or seeing.

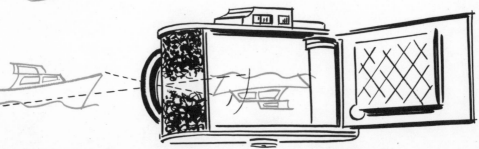

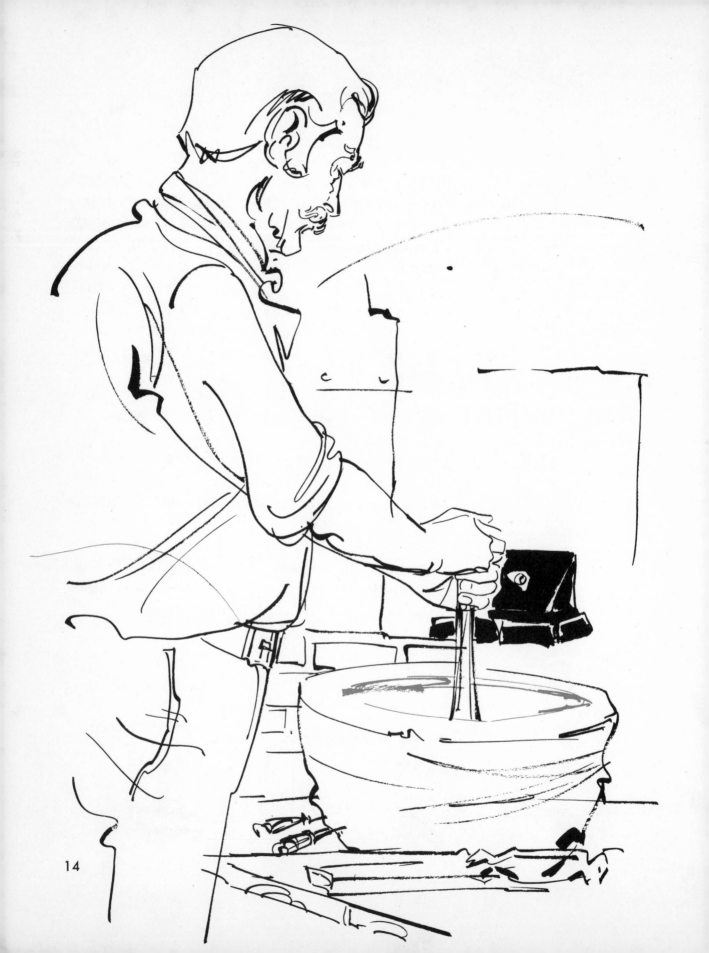

14

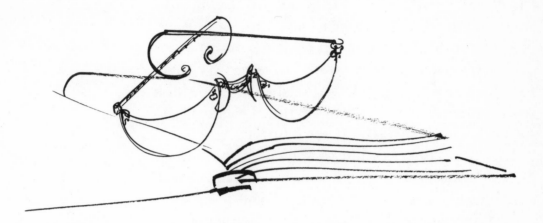

III WHAT EYEGLASSES DO

How Glasses Were Developed

People wear glasses in order to see better. Three children out of every 10 who are of school age wear glasses.

Glasses are made up of a frame that rests on the nose and ears and of lenses cut from clear plastic or a special kind of glass called optical glass.

Optical glass is different from ordinary glass. It must be chemically and physically perfect without bubbles or streaks.

In 1790 a Swiss watchmaker, Pierre-Louis Guinand, discovered a way to make glass without streaks. The Guinand family kept the formula for making optical glass a secret for many years.

Other glassmakers knew that to make glass, sand and certain metals had to be heated in a clay pot over a hot furnace. When the mixture melted, the pot was removed and slowly cooled. Then both pot and the hard glass that had formed were broken up, and selected pieces of glass were softened by heat and pressed into rectangular slabs. The slabs were polished, and the best quality glass was sawed or pressed into lenses or prisms.

But nobody was able to make glass as pure as the Guinands until their secret formula was discovered. The secret was that the glass had to be stirred carefully while it was being cooled. This is how some optical glass is made today.

Glasses are not a new invention. Magnifiers and burning glasses of crystal were known in ancient times. They probably were used even then by old people to help them see close objects. As people get older their lenses become less elastic and cannot thicken enough to accommodate. The magnifying glass, which is a convex lens, can be used to help focus for near vision.

In 1268 Roger Bacon suggested that artificial lenses be used to help people see. We do not know the name of the first person who actually invented spectacles. We do know that Alexander de Spina, who died in the year 1313, reinvented spectacles and is said to be the second inventor. In the 1350's the only spectacles made had convex lenses. Two hundred years later, in 1550, spectacles with concave lenses became available. And in 1785 Benjamin Franklin invented bifocals in which each spectacle glass consists of two lenses, one above the other —a smaller lens for near vision placed below the center of a larger lens which is for distant vision.

Why People Wear Glasses

Most people with glasses wear them because they are nearsighted or farsighted or have astigmatism. Nearsighted people can see best objects that are close to them. Farsighted people have difficulty seeing objects that are close to them and can see best objects that are far away.

Nearsightedness

Distant objects look blurred to nearsighted people because the light rays reflected from the objects are brought to a focus in *front* of the retina instead of on the retina. This may happen if a person's eyes are a little too long from front to back. The lens is too thick, and it bends the light rays too much for the length of the eyeball so that the image comes to a focus before it reaches the retina.

If the nearsighted person holds a book up close to his face, he can read better because the

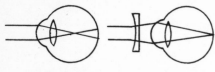

HOW CONCAVE LENS CORRECTS

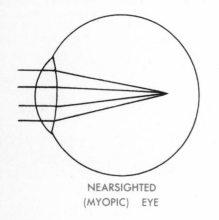

NEARSIGHTED
(MYOPIC) EYE

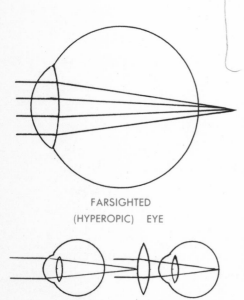

FARSIGHTED
(HYPEROPIC) EYE

HOW CONVEX LENS CORRECTS

light rays become more divergent or spread apart. Then when the lens of his eye bends the light the refraction or bending is not too much, and the image comes to a focus on the retina instead of in front of it.

Concave eyeglass lenses are used to make light rays more divergent before they enter the eye. This helps overcome the converging action of the natural lenses of the nearsighted person's eyes.

Nearsightedness is called *myopia,* meaning shut-eyed or shortsightedness. *My-opia* comes from *myein,* to shut and *opos,* the eye.

Farsightedness

Near objects appear fuzzy to farsighted people because the light rays reflected from the objects are brought to a focus *behind* the retina. The farsighted person's eyes are too short from front to back. The lenses cannot thicken enough to bend the light rays as much as necessary so the image comes to a focus behind the retina.

A farsighted person usually can see an object held at arm's length better than one held in front of his face. The light rays coming from the more distant object are less divergent so that the natural lens does not have to bend them so much.

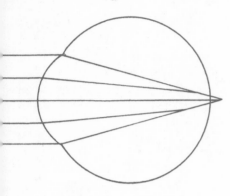

HYPEROPIC ASTIGMATISM

Convex eyeglass lenses are used to bend light rays before they enter the eye. This helps the thin lenses of the farsighted person's eyes bend light rays enough to come to a focus on the retina instead of beyond it.

The medical term for farsightedness is *hyperopia,* meaning fareyedness. *Opia* comes from *opos,* the Greek for eye. *Hyper* is Greek for over or above.

Astigmatism

The word astigmatism comes from *a,* the Greek for not and *stigma,* the prick of a pointed instrument or a spot. It means without a spot or point. In astigmatism light rays do not come to a sharp point on the retina because the curve of the cornea and lens is not even in all directions. Light rays are bent more in one direction than in another so that they come to focus at different spots. This results in an image that is not clear.

Astigmatism is very common. Most people have a little unevenness in curvature of the lens and cornea which they get used to without glasses. When much astigmatism is present, however, eyeglasses are used with the lens curved only in certain directions to correct for the unevenness of the eye. Astigmatism may

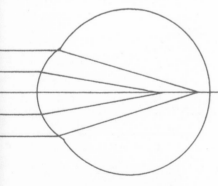

MYOPIC ASTIGMATISM

occur with nearsightedness or farsightedness.

Some amusement parks have astigmatic mirrors. When a person looks in such a mirror, his body appears out of shape.

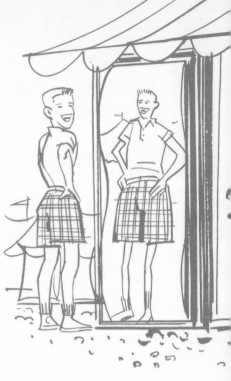

How the Eyes Cooperate

Each eyeball is attached by six muscles to a bony socket or hollow in the skull. These muscles turn the eye out, in, up, down, down and out, up and out, down and in or down and out. If a muscle of one eye pulls harder than the same muscle of the other eye, the two eyes cannot look together at an object. One eye may go up, down, in or out while the other eye stays steady. When the muscles do not work cooperatively as they should, *strabismus* occurs. The common names for strabismus are cross-eye and squint.

When the eyes pull independently instead of together, the image of an object that a person is looking at does not fall on the right spots in the retinas of the two eyes; and the brain cannot fuse or put together these images. At first the person sees two objects instead of one. After a while he learns to block out the image in the turned eye so that he sees only one image with the good eye. If a person uses only one eye for a long time, he may not develop *binocular* or normal two-eyed vision. Without binocular vision we would not be able to tell how far away objects are.

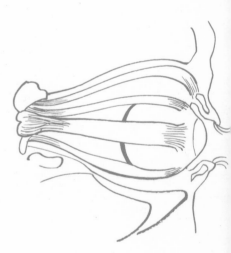

EYE MUSCLES

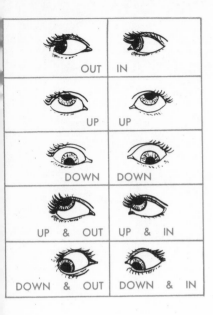

OUT	IN
UP	UP
DOWN	DOWN
UP & OUT	UP & IN
DOWN & OUT	DOWN & IN

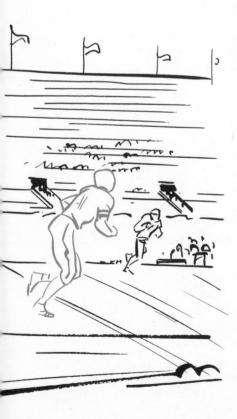

The most common type of strabismus in children is *convergent strabismus* in which the eyes turn in. In *divergent strabismus* the eyes turn out. Convergent strabismus is seen frequently in farsighted children who are trying to accommodate or focus on near objects. With corrective glasses the eyes may straighten out. Sometimes an operation or special exercises are needed to correct squint. Treatment depends on what the eye doctor considers best for each patient.

Contact Lenses

Contact lenses are a special kind of eyeglasses. They are not set in frames and worn outside the eye like ordinary glasses. Instead, they are put directly on the eyeball and are almost invisible. One type of contact lenses fits over the cornea or front part of the eye. Another type fits over the sclera or white of the eye. Contact lenses are helpful in a few very unusual disorders and following certain eye operations. For most eye problems requiring glasses, ordinary spectacles are used.

Sometimes athletes, actors and actresses wear contact lenses when regular eyeglasses would interfere with their work. Although some teen-agers prefer the appearance of contact lenses to regular glasses, in most cases there is no medical reason for their use. In addition, contact lenses are very expensive.

21

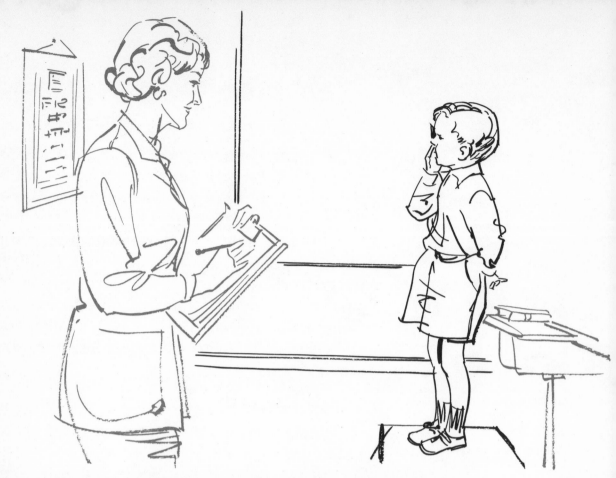

IV EYE TESTING IN SCHOOL

In most schools, beginning with the first grade, the student's eyes are tested by the school nurse.

Although many eye problems begin at birth, some do not appear until school age. The teacher may notice that a pupil blinks or frowns while trying to see the blackboard. Nearsighted students hold their books close to their eyes or keep their heads down close to their desks. Some people who seem to be slow in learning to read actually have trouble seeing.

The Snellen Test

Because so much of what we learn comes through our eyes, most school health programs include a test of *visual acuity*. This is a way of finding out how well a person can see small objects and printed letters and numbers.

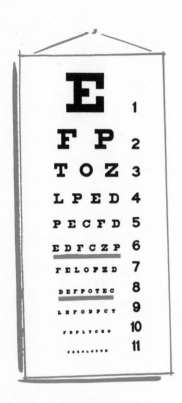

SNELLEN CHART

One hundred years ago, in 1862, Herman Snellen, a Dutch physician, found a simple, accurate way to test sight. The Snellen chart that he made, which is still in use today, consists of pictures, letters and numbers of different sizes. Each symbol is constructed so that it can be seen by a normal eye at a specially marked distance. A letter marked "20" should be seen at a distance of 20 feet. A "100" letter should be seen at 100 feet.

When a person takes the test he is asked to read the smallest letters he can see while 20 feet away from the chart. A distance of 20 feet is chosen because rays of light from this point are practically parallel.

The usual normal reading is 20/20. This is not a fraction but simply a way of stating findings at a given distance. The 20 in the top number is the test distance of 20 feet. The 20 in the bottom number is the "20" letter that normal eyes can see at the test distance. Vision of 20/100 is not 1/5 of normal but simply means that at 20 feet the person reads letters which normally are seen at 100 feet. A reading of 20/100 is a good reason for a person to have a complete eye examination by a doctor. The Snellen test does not diagnose eye disease. It lets one know whether acuity or sharpness of vision is normal.

If the school nurse finds that a student's eyes do not meet the average standard, she will let the parents know so that they can ask a physician to do a complete examination.

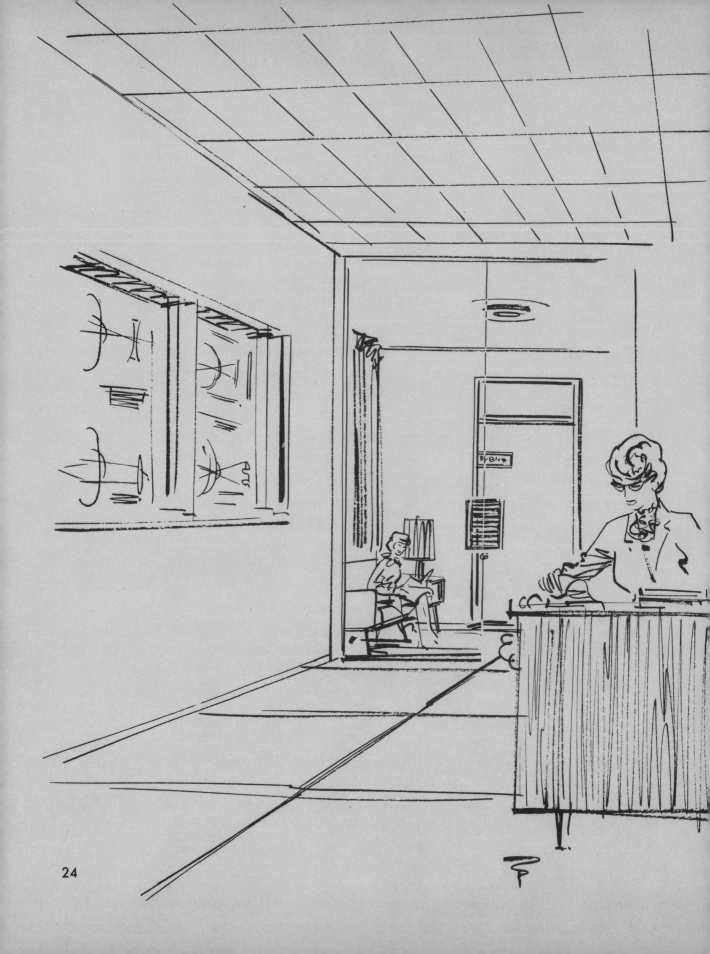

24

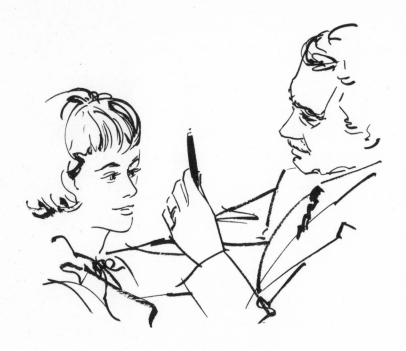

V THE DOCTOR'S OFFICE

The Eye Examination

The first thing the eye doctor usually does is to ask the patient some questions about his health and about his eyes. The next thing the doctor does is to look at the patients eyelids and the front of the eyes. Then he tests the eye muscles to see how well they cooperate. After that he may check visual acuity with the Snellen chart.

When a very young patient is examined, an easy way to measure sight is with the E chart. On this chart the letter E is printed in different sizes and turned in different directions. The child is given a large letter E to hold in his hand. He can turn the letter E that he is holding so that its branches point in the same direction as those of the letter E on the chart.

The Ophthalmoscope

The doctor uses an ophthalmoscope (ophthal-mo-scope) to examine the inside of the eye. Some people say that ophthalmology — the science that includes study and treatment of the eye — can be divided into two periods of history: one, before invention of the ophthalmoscope and two, after invention of the ophthalmoscope. The reason for this is that the ophthalmoscope is so valuable in examining the eye.

Two thousand years ago people thought light was magic that flashed out of the eyes. In the first century a man named Pliny wrote that the eyes of cats, goats and wolves glow at night and give off a light like fire. Many years later, in 1796, Fermin noted the glow of human eyes. In 1810 Benjamin Provost discovered that cats' eyes did not shine in a completely dark room.

In 1851 a young man with a long name, Hermann Ludwig Ferdinand Von Helmholtz, wanted to show his students why most of the time

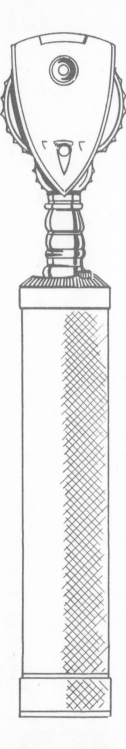

OPHTHALMOSCOPE

the pupil of the eye appears black but some of the time the eye seems to give out a red light.

Helmholtz, who was 29 years old, glued together some pieces of polished glass and cardboard. The glass, acting as a mirror, took light from outside the eye and reflected it into the eye through the pupil. At the same time the glass plates were transparent enough so that Helmholtz could see through them right into the back of the eye. The retina appeared red. Helmholtz showed that the light that comes out of the eye is actually the same light that goes into the eye reflected back to its source.

Hence the cats' eyes and the eyes of man were bright only when light from some source, such as a candle, was shined on them and reflected back to the observer.

While trying to find out what makes the pupil look black or red, Helmholtz invented a useful tool. He wrote his father a letter about his invention, which he called an "egg of Columbus" that had to be handled with great care. Helmholtz's cardboard egg was the beginning of the most important instrument that doctors use today for examining the eye—the ophthalmoscope.

An Englishman, Charles Babbage, invented an ophthalmoscope even before Helmholtz; but physicians did not find out about this until later. With the ophthalmoscope the doctor can look into the eye to find out if there is any disease that interferes with seeing.

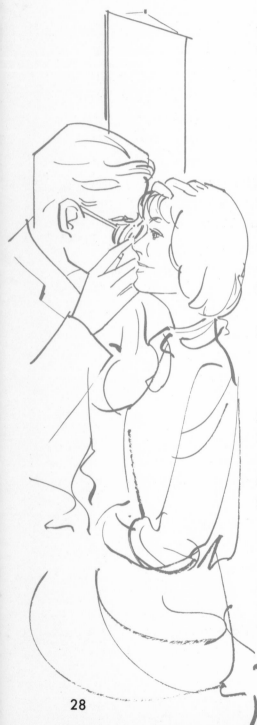

The electric ophthalmoscope of today works better and is easier to use than Helmholtz's original model. It consists of a flashlight handle with a wheel at the top. The wheel or disc contains many lenses varying from weak to strong that can be used to focus on the patient's eye.

Light from the ophthalmoscope shines into the patient's eye and returns to the doctor's eye through a hole in the lens-disc. By turning the disc, the doctor can choose the right lens to help him focus exactly on the structures inside the patient's eye. He can see blood vessels, nerves and other parts of the retina. He also can get some idea as to whether the patient is nearsighted or farsighted.

Examination with the ophthalmoscope often is done in a dark room because the pupils relax and dilate in the dark just as they become wider at night than during the day. With the pupils dilated it is easy to see through them into the eye. Also it is possible to test the pupil's reaction to light. If a bright light shines on the pupil, the normal pupil constricts or becomes smaller. This contraction of the pupil in response to light is called the *pupillary reflex*.

Eyedrops

Frequently *eyedrops* are used during the examination. Their effect lasts from a few hours to three weeks depending upon the type of drug used. During that time the patient's vision will be fuzzy. For very young children the mother may be given the drops to put in the child's eyes at home before returning to the doctor's office. For older children and adults drops are put in the eyes at the doctor's office.

Eyedrops work two ways. First, they dilate the pupils so that the inside of the eye can be seen better. Second, eyedrops temporarily paralyze or knock out the ciliary muscles. With the ciliary muscles blocked, the lens remains flat and does not accommodate. This may help the doctor to measure the amount of incorrect refraction or light bending of the eye.

When the doctor has completed the examination and knows whether the patient is nearsighted or farsighted, has astigmatism, strabismus or some other eye disorder, he can decide if eyeglasses will be helpful.

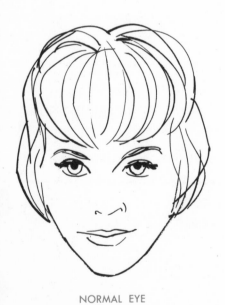

NORMAL EYE

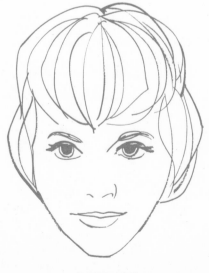

DILATED EYE

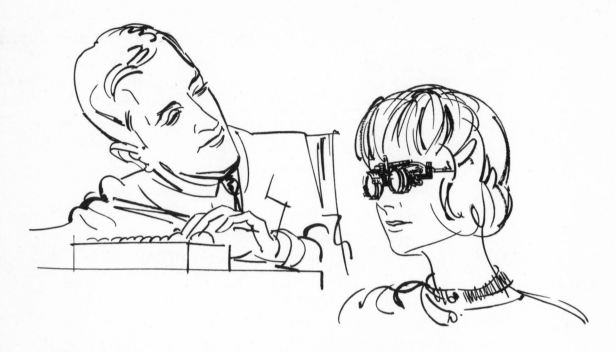

VI GETTING GLASSES

After the eye doctor has decided that spectacles will be helpful, he finds out what kind of glass lens is best for the patient. This measurement for glasses is called *refraction* because it has to do with the bending or refracting of light rays.

The doctor keeps a supply of trial lenses in his office. He puts different lenses in a frame that fits over the patient's eyes. The Snellen test for sharpness of vision may be repeated with the artificial lenses in place. The doctor chooses the lens that will make the patient's vision as normal as possible.

An *ophthalmologist* is a medical doctor. He has had special training to diagnose and treat all disorders of the eyes in addition to examining them for glasses. *Oculist* is another name for ophthalmologist.

An *optometrist* has had special training to prescribe and fit eyeglasses for such disorders as nearsightedness, farsightedness and astigmatism.

An *optician* can fill the patient's prescription for eyeglasses by grinding lenses and fitting them into a frame. He also sells other optical instruments such as telescopes and binoculars.

Why Glasses?

The eye is a very complicated and very wonderful structure. By enabling us to see, it makes it possible for us to learn about people, about the world, about much of life. Our eyes are so important to us that when they do not work well we should see a medical doctor. He can find out what is wrong, and many times eyeglasses are just what we need.

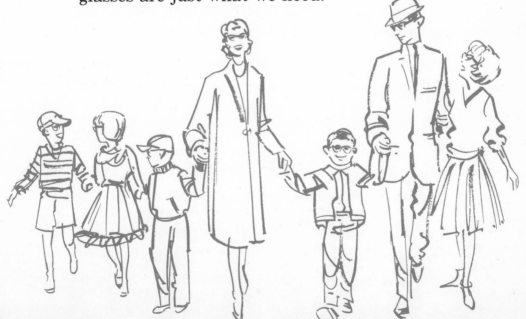

We specialize in publishing quality books for
young people. For a complete list please write
LERNER PUBLICATIONS COMPANY
241 First Avenue North, Minneapolis, Minnesota 55401